Love Yourself, so…

Hate the Weight!

LOSING WEIGHT is not just a cosmetic change; it can give you the sense of being in better control of your health and life.

This compact volume provides many wise tips on how to slim down naturally and effectively.

Clearly written by one who has been there, it will help you avoid the pitfalls on the way to the slimmer body you've been looking for.

Neal Barnard, M.D.

President
Physicians Committee for Responsible Medicine
510 Wisconsin Avenue #404
Washington, D.C. 20016

Love Yourself, so...

Hate the Weight!

Brother Craig
(Who lost 114 pounds in 14 months.)

100 Diet, Metabolic-Rate-Enhancing and Exercise Tips That Really Work!

Photographs:

Front cover, back cover ("After"): *Robert Mayer*
Back cover ("Before"): *Richard Rotondi*
Text illustrations: *Brother John; p. 12, Robert Mayer*

Woodbridge Press • Santa Barbara, California 93102

Important Notice: This book presents information that was effective and helpful for Brother Craig. You should *consult your physician as to whether it is appropriate to your personal needs.*

Published and distributed by

Woodbridge Press Publishing Company, Santa Barbara, California 93102

Printed in the United States of America.

Distributed simultaneously in Canada, The United Kingdom, Australia, New Zealand and The Republic of South Africa.

Library of Congress Cataloging-in-Publication Data:

Craig, Brother
    Love yourself, so . . . hate the weight : 100 diet, metabolic-rate-enhancing and exercise tips that really work! / Brother Craig.
        p.   cm.
        "Photographs: front cover, back cover ("After"): Robert Mayer. Back cover ("Before"): Richard Rotondi. Text illustrations: Brother John; p. 12, Robert Mayer."
        Includes bibliographical references (p.   ).
        ISBN 0-88007-215-6 (alk. paper)
        1. Weight loss. I. Title
    RM222.2.C714   1996
    613.2'5—dc20   96-34357
                                                            CIP

To all the people who called me fatso, blimpo, husky, stout, rotund, circular, big, and a little on the chubby side: thank you for caring.

Brother Craig

And God said, "Behold, I have given you every plant yielding seed which is upon the face of all the earth, and every tree with seed in its fruit; you shall have them for food."

The Bible (Genesis 1:29)

Foreword

My weight was 237 pounds. Fourteen months later, it was 123 pounds. This book tells you how *I lost 114 pounds*—and how you (or someone you love if you are already slim) can lose weight, too, whether it's 114 pounds or just 14 pounds.

As you begin a new, renewing lifestyle (and that's really what this program was for me), be enthusiastic about it. Encourage your sense of humor. Laugh. Find fun with friends and laughter, not food.

Eat to stay healthy, to be alive, to be strong and have energy. Do not eat for emotional reasons. (Sure, that's been on all the talk shows—but it's true.)

The psychological basis of this metabolic-enhancing diet and exercise program is that you *hate* your (over)weight.

If you don't hate it, work on that. *Hate it a lot.* There is lots of bad hate in the world. We don't want any of that. I'm not advocating self-hate.

I agree with Dr. Dean Ornish, the expert on reversing heart disease, that *you* are not the same as your *weight*. So hating the weight isn't the same as hating yourself.

But do hate the weight—that excessive, life-diminishing weight. Love yourself; love food a little less. There is more to life than just the special foods you now like. (Train those taste buds!!!)

And what about better looks, more energy and just feeling better about life in general?!

I hope all these benefits will really, *really* motivate you to get rid of those unneeded pounds! I know I really, yes, extremely wanted to be more slim and healthy.

This was not an extreme program for me in any sense of being unhealthful. Losing 114 pounds in 14 months means I lost less than two pounds per week. That is a modest rate of loss.

But just think. Even at that rate, three months from now you could be 25 pounds lighter, or in a couple of months, 16 pounds—in less than six months you could slim down by 50 pounds if you need to.

So hate the weight!

And pray. Ask God to help you. He will. Show Him that you really want to lose weight by really trying. And show yourself, too. The Lord loves a cheerful giver—so give up some weight cheerfully!

Let me know how you do. Send me your ideas. Good luck and God bless you!

I would like to thank all the people who helped me with this book; especially Joshua Paulin who typed the manuscript, Brother John and Edward Driscoll for their editing, and Elizabeth Ann Paulin, my writing teacher, for her help and encouragement.

And a special "Thank you" to Dr. Neal Barnard for his kind recommendation.

Brother Craig

Some good advice about food choices.

This book encourages what is called a "vegan" diet (say "*vee'* gun"). That means no animal foods; for example, meat, fish, poultry, eggs and dairy foods. Consult you own health advisors, but from my own experience, I really believe in this diet—for weight loss, for optimum health.

And I recommend that you choose organically produced foods as consistently as you can. Organically grown foods are more healthful for you, not only because they are free from chemical pesticides, but also, I believe, they are more nutritious, because pesticides destroy some of a food's nutrients.

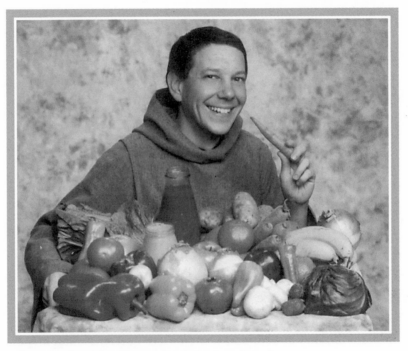

Lose weight and still enjoy foods in abundance!

Vegans are encouraged to take a vitamin B_{12} supplement, since it is found mainly in dairy products and meat and only in very small amounts in some products like wheat grass and barley green. Nutritional authority John Robbins (*Diet for a New America.* Walpole, NH: Stillpoint) recommends this supplement and gives preference to the sublingual form. He recommends an adult dose of 2 mcg per day (that's not milligrams—*micrograms*—microgram is also written μg).

Vitamin B_{12} can also be purchased as a nasal gel. Dr. Earl Mindell, one of America's most respected nutritional authorities, says that B_{12} seems to be absorbed better when used as a gel than when taken orally. He also indicates that B vitamins, including B_{12}, are absorbed better in the body when combined with calcium. (*Dr. Earl Mindell's Live Longer and Feel Better with Vitamins and Minerals.* New Canaan, CT: Keats.)

Many of the authors cited in this book for good information of various kinds present dietary suggestions that are not in the vegan mode, and perhaps would not even advocate it. I can simply tell you that for me it has been an excellent dietary program.

For further information about the healthfulness of a vegan diet you could read *Vegan Nutrition: Pure and Simple*, by Michael Klaper, M.D. (Umatilla, FL: Gentle World, Inc.) Your bookstore could order it, or write: P.O. Box 1418, Umatilla, FL 32784.

Here they are:

*100 valuable tips, pointers,
insights and encouragements.*

1. Hate the weight.

The first step to weight loss is to hate the weight. The second step is to pray to God for help. I mean it. Pray to be strong; to really do it this time. The third step is to make your diet-exercise program the first thing in your life. From now on it must be your main concern. Nothing must be allowed to take you away from it. No faltering. No excuses!

2. When you lose, you win.

Losing weight will give you only benefits. Your health will improve. Your looks will improve. Your attitudes, emotions, everything will improve. You'll be a new you—fully alive. I have even heard that overweight people are less likely to be hired for a job and less apt to be promoted. So you could even discover new financial success, new job satisfaction.

3. Eat strawberries.

Only 26 calories in half a cup. (I'm going to give you some very simple, attractive ideas like this along the way—not just heavy[!] advice.) Strawberries have three times the vitamin C that oranges have. Also, those little red berries have more potassium and more fiber than whole wheat bread.

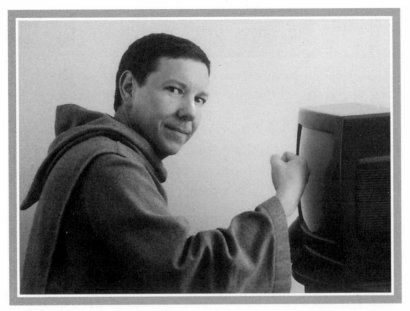

Control that TV! It's hard (impossible?) for couch potatoes to lose weight!

4. Get up. Get going.

Lose weight. Keep moving. Keep busy. Forget food. Turn off the T.V. Take brisk walks. Go out. Be active.

The more active you are, the more calories you'll burn. I agree with best-selling motivational authors and speakers Mark Victor Hansen and Jack Canfield (*Dare to Win.* New York: Berkley) that being fit is fun and that the discipline of eating right, consistently, is actually enjoyable. (Busy as they are, these speakers run five days a week.)

5. *Weight loss, exercise— you just can't separate them.*

Besides weight loss, exercise does lots of other good things for you. It increases the supply of oxygen to your brain, for example. It also causes a release of mood-elevating brain chemicals called endorphins, according to biochemist and fitness authority Covert Bailey. These endorphins can have a mood-elevating effect. They are the body's natural pain killer. You'll think better and be happier.

Moderately intense exercise for about a half-hour—if you are physically fit, or as directed by your health or fitness counselor— causes the maximum "high" because it causes the greatest release of endorphins into the bloodstream.

Exercise gives your body more oxygen. Oxygen burns up calories. Make your exercise time fun. Invite a friend. If the weather is bad go to the mall and walk briskly.

Relax when you exercise—don't hold your breath. Before and after exercising drink plenty of water.

6. Exercise increases your metabolic rate —which burns calories!

As Covert Bailey explains in *The Fit or Fat Woman* (New York: Houghton Mifflin), moderate exercise speeds up one's metabolic rate (intense exercise slows it down!!!), and the benefit continues even after exercising. Short intense exercise burns up carbohydrates. Longer, moderate exercise uses the fat that's stored in the muscles.

7. Begin a new life today.

Start losing weight today and you can begin to really live today! It's true.

We sometimes try in vain to solve our life problems without considering health and weight at all. Still, we know that being overweight can cause lots of problems—emotional, psychological, physiological and financial problems (a heart bypass?).

Having your body in shape—fit and slim—benefits your mind. It benefits your soul, makes you feel like being kinder, more charitable, more inclined to pray, to practice virtue. It really does.

8. Be well—don't be ill.

Being overweight can lead to or intensify a lot of diseases: diabetes, osteoarthritis, coronary heart disease, gout, for example. It can also increase cholesterol and triglyceride levels and blood pressure— even shorten your life. A diet high in fat can also increase the risk of cancer, according to nutritionists and dietitians Annette B. Natow and Jo-Ann Heslin, in *The Fat Attack* (New York: Pocket Books).

9. Eat breakfast!

Don't skip it. I can tell you from personal experience that breakfast boosts energy and makes me feel better. You may have observed, as I have, that people who skip breakfast often make up the calories by eating more later in the day!

(Thinking of early morning, many people like to exercise then. But remember that muscles are less limber so extra warming up, perhaps a hot shower, then slow jogging in place and then gentle stretching before you exercise, really helps.)

10. 'Don't eat fattening foods! Don't do it!'

That should be emblazoned on your refrigerator and your food cabinets (although, really, there shouldn't be any fattening foods in the house!). When you go out always carry low-calorie, fat-free food with you—so you won't turn to high-calorie or high-fat food as snacks.

11. *You will lose weight.*

If you do all the things I mention here, my personal experience tells me you will lose weight! If it doesn't seem to be working, please check to see which part you've omitted, or neglected.

(And, of course, be sure your health advisor says you can do all these things.)

12. *Walk. Walk briskly.*

It is really a very good exercise. Walk as briskly as your present condition permits. As you become more fit, you can walk even more briskly. Hand-held weights (again, appropriate to your size and state of fitness) make it even better.

Walking also relieves stress and tension—fewer excuses to eat!

Walking in sand or freshly plowed earth burns more calories, because it's harder.

Walking uphill burns even more calories.

Going upstairs increases the burning of calories still more.

Brisk walking reduces bad cholesterol (LDL) and raises the level of good cholesterol (HDL) as does all good exercise.

Doctors, studies and the media are telling us that exercise can help to increase the ratio of "good" HDL cholesterol to "bad" LDL cholesterol.

So go for a walk, now! You can read the rest of this later.

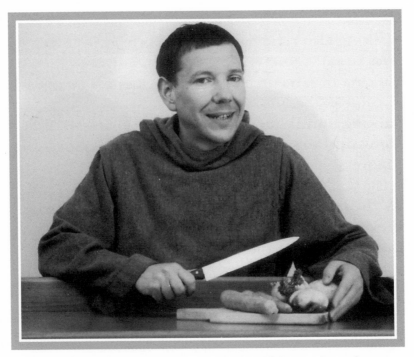

If "trim" is what you want, use that knife on delicious, low-calorie veggies!

13. Eat low calorie foods

And especially very low fat foods. Every gram of fat has nine calories. Every gram of carbohydrates or protein has only four.

Various authorities say that at least 20 percent of the calories eaten as carbohydrates and protein are used up by the body as it processes them! But as the body processes fat, only three percent of the calories are used up! Basically, then, the fat you eat becomes fat on you. No fair! But it's true.

According to Dr. Dean Ornish (*Eat More, Weigh Less.* New York: HarperCollins), you need only about four to six percent of your calories as fat in order to get the essential fatty acids, although his "Life Choice" diet suggests about 10 percent for a comfortable margin.

14. Lies, myths and tragic errors:

1. Diets don't work. (They do.)
2. Diets don't work because when you go off them you gain the weight back. (This statement proves that diets do work and that going off them doesn't work!)
3. You've got to accept being fat. (You don't!)
4. Losing weight won't make you happier. (It will!)

15. Your stomach doesn't say, 'You're hungry!' Your brain does.

It takes 15 to 20 minutes for the brain to know you are full, so eat slowly; leave the table, wait to eat more. Also, chew well—it greatly helps your digestion.

But when you really are hungry here's a low-calorie suggestion—have low-fat, healthy bran cereal or another low-fat, healthy cereal. Use unsweetened apple juice instead of milk. Do it. (You can find this juice as frozen concentrate or ready-to-use in bottles.) And don't expect this cereal to taste like "cereal and milk." It's different. Enjoy it for what it actually is.

16. Asparagus sandwich, anyone?

Here's one of my favorite recipes. So simple. An asparagus sandwich. Now asparagus is quite expensive, so skip going out to eat and have this instead. You will come out saving money:

Two slices of diet whole wheat bread. (35-40 calories per slice).

A cup of asparagus, steamed (104 calories) or pressure-cooked. This sandwich has only 170-180 calories!

A steamed or pressure-cooked spinach sandwich is

great also. Add thinly sliced raw onions and mustard to either sandwich, if you wish. Enjoy!

If you have any real experience with dieting you already know that unusual foods like this can be truly attractive—at a small cost in calories.

(Steaming is the best way to cook veggies because it lets them retain more nutrients. Microwaving and pressure cooking are also good.)

17. Exercise!

There. I said it again. Please do it. Make time for two half-hour sessions a day.

Do whatever your state of physical fitness permits. See a health or physical fitness professional.

Aerobics, such as jogging, biking, brisk walking,

burns calories. Brisk walking can burn the same number of calories as jogging but you must do it longer. Lift weights *after* doing your aerobics since that builds more muscle than doing it before.

Lifting weights (mindful of your present state of fitness) will make you stronger. With greater muscle strength you'll be able, in time, to do more aerobics.

Before doing your actual aerobic workout, jog slowly in place for 5 to 10 minutes, to warm up.

Then do some stretching. Stretch before and after your workout—gently stretch your legs, arms, etc. Doing this before your workout limbers you up for the workout. Stretching afterward makes the muscles more flexible for the next workout.

Fitness expert Edward J. Jackowski (*Hold It! You're Exercising Wrong!* New York: Fireside) praises stretching as the most important part of a workout.

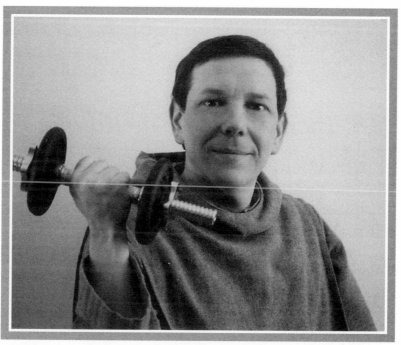

Weights in your hands can help to reduce weight elsewhere!

Stretching improves mechanical efficiency and increases the flow of blood to your muscles. This makes exercise easier and reduces the risk of injury.

18. *Increase your metabolic rate.*

In moderation, and if they agree with you, onions, hot mustard and hot peppers actually increase your metabolic or calorie-burning rate! And coffee, too. But again, in moderation.

I ate no meat, fish, poultry, eggs, dairy products. Foods like these increase your metabolic rate only a very tiny bit.

Alcohol actually does decrease, yes, it slows down, your metabolic rate.

19. *It's not easy, but you can do it.*

Fitness guru Richard Simmons says that. I say it, too. Believe him. *Believe me, too.*

20. *Never go off your diet.*

No exceptions! Not weddings, holidays, vacations, depression, problems, etc. Before you go to a special event (where there may be unhealthful, fattening food) have a big salad at home first.

21. *Eat more, very small meals*

... of very low calorie food—rather than a few larger ones. Frequent eating keeps your metabolic rate up. Snack all day! To lose weight, I ate about 9-12 times each day. (The only problem was that I had to brush my teeth more often than I used to! After every meal, you know.)

The New England Journal of Medicine reported in October 1989, a study by Dr. David Jenkins, University of Toronto. Two groups of people ate exactly the same kinds and amount of food. But one group ate it in three meals each day; the other in seventeen snacks each day.

The second group lowered their cholesterol by 15 percent and had more stable blood sugar levels, making energy levels more constant. Their bodies produced less insulin, which is good because when your body produces *more* insulin, more fat goes from your blood stream to your cells—making you fatter.

Here are some great low-calorie foods:

> Apples: 66 calories, 4 oz.; 80 calories, one medium apple.
> Asparagus: 13 calories, 4 spears or 2 oz.
> Bagels: some plain or onion ones are only 150 calories each.
> Beans: 115 calories, ½ cup cooked. Most legumes; that is, beans, such as navy, black, chickpea (garbanzo), have from 115 to 130 calories in ½ cup cooked.

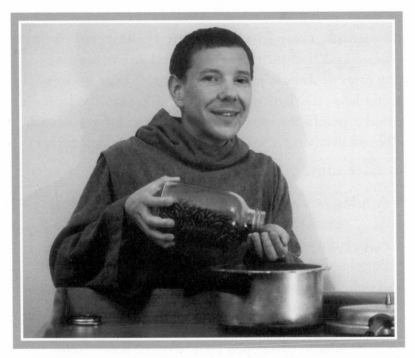

Beans are a wonder-food, nutritious (including quality protein), with few calories.

Bell peppers: 12 calories, ½ cup raw.

Berries: 50 calories, ½ cup raw.

Broccoli: 12 calories, ½ cup raw (23 calories, ½ cup cooked).

Brussels sprouts: 20 calories, ½ cup raw (30 calories, ½ cup cooked).

Buckwheat: 100 calories, ½ cup cooked.

Bulgur: 120 calories, ½ cup cooked.

Cabbage: 16 calories, ½ cup cooked.

Carrots: 24 calories, ½ cup raw (35 calories, ½ cup cooked); or 1 medium carrot, 20 calories.

Cauliflower: 12 calories, ½ cup raw (15 calories, ½ cup cooked).

Chickpeas: 135 calories ½ cup cooked.

Chili peppers: 30 calories, ½ cup.

Garlic: 4 calories per clove.

Grapefruit: 44 calories per ½ cup.

Greens: 8 calories, ½ cup raw (16 calories, ½ cup cooked).

Leeks: 8 calories, ½ cup cooked.

Lentils: 115 calories, ½ cup cooked.

Lettuce: 8 calories, 1 cup.

Melons: 26 calories, ½ cup.

Millet: 50 calories, ½ cup cooked.

Onions: 27 calories, ½ cup raw.

Oranges: 67 calories, 5 oz.

Papaya: 118 calories, 1 lb.

Peaches: 36 calories, 3 oz.

Potatoes: 155 calories, 5 oz. baked (125 calories, 5 oz. boiled).

Soybeans: 150 calories, ½ cup cooked.

Spinach: 6 calories, ½ cup raw (20 calories, ½ cup cooked).

Sprouts: 10 calories, 1 cup raw.
Tomatoes: 24 calories, 4 oz. raw.
Whole wheat bread, diet type: 40 calories,
    1 slice.

22. *Develop a fear of eating fat!*

Don't believe advertising on the front label of a product; read the back! Terms like "lean" and "low fat" are often misleading. They usually refer to the percentage of fat in relation to the weight of the serving. Hey, what can one potato chip weigh?

Warning! Warning! Here's the big problem—85 percent fat-free means 85 percent of the weight is fat-free. Example: one hot dog has 90 calories with 7 grams of fat. Figure it out: 1g fat = 9 calories; so it has 9 x 7 = 63 calories as fat. Thus—about 70 percent of the total calories are from fat!

Remember: 85 percent fat-free in this case means it contains 70 percent fat in terms of calories! Call the FDA!!! "Extra lean" ground beef has 54 percent of its calories from fat.

Dr. Dean Ornish believes that scientific evidence increasingly associates diets high in animal fat with chances of heart disease, breast cancer in women, osteoporosis, stroke, diabetes, gallbladder disease, hypertension—all among the diseases that take the greatest toll in our society.

Dr. Neal Barnard, president of the Physicians Committee for Responsible Medicine and author of several books on healthy eating, says emphatically that vegetarian foods are the winners when it comes to weight control. (*Foods that Cause You To Lose Weight—the Negative Calorie Effect*. McKinney, TX: The Magni Group.)

Here are some no-calorie foods. Well, almost.

Most mustards (not Dijon) and dill pickles have less than 5 calories per serving which allows their labels to read 0 calories.

Cucumbers have hardly any calories and make a great sandwich with whole wheat bread. Lettuce is another almost calorie-free food. Eat green lettuce; the white is almost nutrient-free.

Eating just a little bit of fat-filled foods, high calorie sweets will only make you want to have more. So . . . avoid them completely!!!

23. Re-educate your 'tastes.'

Learn to do without "tasty" foods like potato chips. Eat delicious foods—veggies, whole wheat bread and raw carrots!

Avoid all cakes, cookies, sweets.

Eat apples, pears, bananas, but no grapes, plums or raisins—all are high-calorie foods because of their high sugar content.

Learn to like foods garnished with herbs and spices (no calories) and vinegar (no calories).

You can change a sweet-tooth into a spicy and tart one by eating raw onions, garlic, mustard and salsa sauce. I know. I did it.

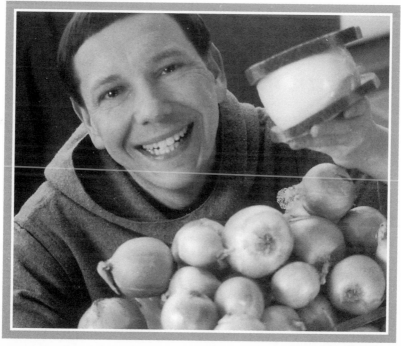

Onions are so good in a diet, you may want to make big, big sandwiches. Kidding!

24. Take a multivitamin-with-minerals tablet each day.

My own diet includes 500 to 800 mg of supplementary calcium and 250-400 mg of supplementary magnesium each day—since I'm not drinking milk or eating other dairy foods. (Besides being fattening, dairy products can contain antibiotics, hormones and pesticides.)

Soy milk is a good source of protein—use the fat-free or low-fat version.

Again, in matters of diet, especially in special conditions like pregnancy, nursing an infant, patients with osteoporosis and so on, be sure to consult your doctor or other qualified health professionals.

25. *Don't let excess weight make you cancer-prone.*

In *The Fat Attack*, by Dr. Annette B. Natow and Jo-Ann Heslin (New York: Pocket Books), I was amazed and saddened to read that evidence links overweight and a high-fat diet—independently—to greater risk of certain cancers.

I also read that overweight causes a person to be almost three times as likely to become diabetic. The risk of diabetes becomes greater as overweight increases.

26. Never eat nuts!

No peanuts—filled with calories from fat and saturated fat. (Okay, peanuts are really legumes, not
nuts.) All other nuts have *more* fat than peanuts.

About fats in general, remember what Covert
Bailey says—the fat you eat today, you will be
"wearing" tomorrow.

27. Develop resistance to fattening foods.

Fattening foods: meat, poultry, fish, eggs, milk,
cheese, yogurt, ice cream, cake, cookies and avocados.

Eat baked potatoes: 155 calories, 5 oz. baked

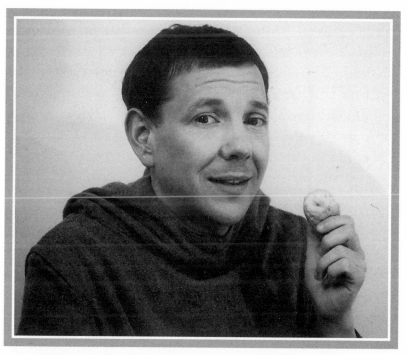

If you're experienced in dieting, you know how delicious even simple foods can be!

(125 calories boiled). Potatoes are not fattening, and if you also eat the skins they are very nutritious. Eat baked potatoes, or steamed, or microwaved (make a slit or they may explode!).

Do eat the skins of potatoes; just underneath are the most nutrients. If you find you can't eat the skin of some potatoes, you may be able to eat that of well scrubbed, thin-skinned "new potatoes."

Low-Cal, Fat-Free, Baked-Potato Topping:

- Mustard or salsa
- Chopped raw onions
- Black pepper and chopped chives
- Fat-free tomato sauce
- Fat-free soy milk
- Mashed butternut squash (sounds crazy but it's really good!)

28. *Don't satisfy your hunger with fat.*

When you're hungry, remember that every gram of fat has 9 calories, every gram of carbohydrates only 4!

Eat complex carbohydrates like brown rice, whole grains like wheat or oats (steel cut are more nutritious than rolled), and veggies.

Carbohydrates enhance your metabolism, according to Dr. Neal Barnard, in his book, *Foods That Cause You to Lose Weight—the Negative Calorie Effect*. (McKinney, TX: The Magni Group). That's what we need to hear!!!

Dr. Barnard goes on to explain that carbohydrates in the body are transformed into various sugars that stimulate the release of insulin. That triggers the production of norepinephrine and thyroid hormone (T3), two natural hormones that increase the metabolic rate. Thus calories are burned more effectively.

Since meat, fish, poultry, eggs and dairy products have virtually no complex carbohydrates, filling up on them makes no sense if you want to lose weight!

That's one reason Dr. Bernard emphasizes that vegetarian menus are the most effective ones in weight control programs.

Plant foods have the added advantage of containing fiber. Grain, beans and veggies contain fiber—makes them filling and satisfying. Again from Dr. Barnard, we learn that a plant-based diet, with its carbohydrates and fiber (which animal products lack), tends to promote slim bodies; animal products tend to produce overweight bodies.

29. *Be aware of the different kinds of fat.*

Let's look at them. There are saturated, polyunsaturated and monounsaturated fats. Actually all fats are really some combination of these with one predominating.

Saturated fat. Stays solid even at room temperature: meat, milk, cheese, butter, coconut, palm and palm-kernel oil and cacao butter. (Hey, folks, how does milk stay solid at room temperature? Anyway, the experts say it's a saturated fat so who am I to argue? Okay, so it contains butterfat which, churned out, becomes butter.)

Saturated fat increases "bad" cholesterol (or LDL—

low-density lipids) in the bloodstream. Hydrogenated and partially hydrogenated fats are vegetable oils that have been made firmer (*e.g.*, corn oil made into margarine.) The result is the same as saturated fat; that is, it raises LDL cholesterol.

Polyunsaturated fat. Stays liquid at room temperature: vegetable oils such as corn, safflower, sunflower and soybean oils. These reduce both "bad" (LDL) and "good" cholesterol (HDL—high density lipids)!

Monounsaturated fat. Liquid at room temperature, but may become solid when cold—such oils as olive, peanut and canola. The big news that I learned from Susan Powter is that one tablespoon of olive oil contains 1.9 grams of saturated fat and canola, .8 gram!

Although these monounsaturated fats are the least damaging in regard to your cholesterol levels, they do contain cholesterol-producing saturated fat.

(What should your total cholesterol level be? Dr. Dean Ornish says 150!)

And all these oils have many calories! One tablespoon of olive oil has 120 calories—all from fat!!!

Even if you eliminated all butter, oils, etc., you would still get enough fat in the vegetable foods you eat that contain some fat.

Dr. Neal Barnard believes that the small amount of fat contained naturally in grains, legumes and vegetables is all that is really needed.

30. What to put on your toast?

Sugar-laden jam or jelly? No way!

Sugar-free jam? No! The sugar-free versions that have fruit sugar for sweetener can contain as many as 12 calories in one tiny teaspoonful.

Rather, use unsweetened applesauce—it has only 50 calories for whole half cup! Or put some mashed bananas on your bread. Seriously, it's great! You ate mashed bananas as a babe-in-arms, didn't you?

31. Read those labels.

It bears repeating. Products can be advertised (on the front) as having "No Fat"; but the side-panel can reveal that the product may have up to 5 grams of fat per serving—even saturated fat—and it can still say "No Fat" on the front of the label.

32. Worried about getting enough protein?

Better you should worry about getting too much!

Gary and Steve Null (*The Complete Handbook of Nutrition.* New York: Dell), point out that a high-protein diet results in phosphorus deficiency. Dr. Andrew Weil (*Natural Health, Natural Medicine.* New York: Houghton Mifflin) tells us that a high protein intake produces a diuretic effect that leaches minerals from the body. Those minerals include calcium, and calcium loss can favor the development of osteoporosis.

Okay, you do need some protein. But not a lot.

John Robbins believes that scientific studies so far indicate that protein need be only about eight percent of your calorie intake; or, according to some studies, even somewhat less.

Dr. Dean Ornish maintains that it is difficult to get too little protein if you eat a variety of foods. Even foods such as whole wheat, oatmeal and pumpkin have protein, meaning they have some of the 28 amino acids that make up protein. That's good.

To get complete protein you could try a little protein complementation two or three times a week, combining different foods with different amino acids.

Legumes are a great help for this. Navy beans or other beans, like black, garbanzo, etc., are a good source of protein. If you use them in combination with grains, you get a more complete protein.

For more help with this, read *David Scott's Protein-Balanced Vegetarian Cookery* (Sebasapol, CA: CRCS Publications).

Soybeans (or tofu made from soybean curd) are a good source of almost-complete protein in themselves. Try a low-fat version of tofu—Mori-Nu Lite is one—found at most large health food stores.

33. Again—exercise! Use those big muscles.

The best fat-burning exercises are those that use big muscles, especially the thigh muscles.

The following exercises burn about the same amount of calories:

Brisk walking: 40 minutes
Bike riding: 20 minutes
Jogging: 15 minutes
Cross-country skiing: 12 minutes

Listen to this—it may help to motivate you not to eat high-calorie or high-fat foods: it takes 30 minutes of moderate aerobic dancing to burn off 12 to 16 corn chips; 40 minutes running at a 10-minutes-a-mile pace to burn off a hot fudge sundae; 30 minutes of racquetball to burn off a slice of blueberry pie!

34. Write things down.

Not only what you eat but how you exercise. (That will be twice a day.)

Best exercises for weight loss?

1. Jumping rope.
2. Cross country skiing.
3. Full court basketball.
4. Approximately equal: squash, handball, paddle ball, racquetball, running, backpacking, hiking, soccer, aerobics and cycling.

(Always be sure that your exercise is appropriate to your level of fitness.)

35. Dance, dance, dance!

Play music you like (lively music: jazz, country, whatever) and dance away the fat!

Or watch videos of old movies while you exercise or while you use a treadmill. It will distract you into doing more!

36. Do gentle
stretching exercises.

Both before and after you exercise. Before, to limber up. After, to prepare your muscles for the next time.

Do stretching at other times, too, when you want to limber up. Relieves tension and you'll feel great. Stretching, I think, is the most enjoyable form of exercise. It makes us supple. It makes us feel good. Check your library for books and videos about stretching.

The basic rules—be gentle, don't bounce or strain, hold the stretch for at least 30 seconds—don't hold your breath! A hot shower or bath, or a sauna or steam bath before you do your stretching will warm up your muscles and increase your flexibility.

An excellent book on stretching is *Staying Flexible—The Full Range of Motion* (Alexandria, VA: Time-Life Books), produced by a team of experts in physical fitness and dance. It is now out of print. Try your library.

Stretching is said to decrease the chance of aches and pains; it helps prevent tendinitis, helps muscle function and performance, protects your back and spine, helps lower blood pressure, stabilizes your heart rate, aids full range of motion and reduces the risk of injury.

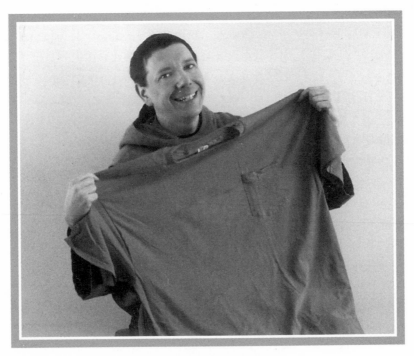

It's hard to believe my old XX Large T-shirts!

37. You'll soon start looking for smaller-size clothes!

I used to buy XX Large T-shirts. I could now sell them as tents.

The other day I went into a store to buy some jeans. Not one pair was small enough—it used to be that I couldn't find a pair large enough. In another store I couldn't find a T-shirt small enough.

A kind clerk suggested I try the boys' department. I bought one there and it's big for me. Those experiences made it all worthwhile!!!

38. You are on a special diet.

So tell your friends that you're on a special diet.

This is very important. If you just say you're on a diet, you'll have to endure: "Oh, just a little bit." "It's not fattening." "I made it just for you." "But it's Christmas" (or Thanksgiving or Happy Tuesday or any excuse). "You have to eat something. This is only 3,500 calories an ounce."

Don't let anyone (not even yourself!) talk you into eating anything you know you shouldn't. Tell people you're on a special diet. You are.

39. Put a picture of a slim person on your refrigerator.

Keep reminding yourself of your goal.

My brother encouraged himself to lose weight by putting up two photos: himself, taken at different times, both slim and heavy. He was helped a lot to stay on his diet by looking at the photos and asking himself, "Which do I want?"

He is now slim and fit—runs 50 miles a week.

40. Warning: sugar everywhere!

Do you know that one 8-ounce glass of orange juice has the juice, sugar and calories of three medium-size oranges! Remember when you are dieting—sugar is sugar is sugar (honey is very high in calories, too). Sugar causes fat retention—makes fat stay on. It also spoils your appetite for eating healthier food.

Clinical nutritionist Cliff Sheats (*Lean Bodies*. New York: Warner), tells us that simple sugars are easily converted into body fat. This is because they are released rapidly into the blood, causing an increase in sugar concentration. This triggers the pancreas to release insulin. Insulin activates fat cell enzymes that help fat traveling in the blood stream to be stored in fat cells. It also prevents glucagon (a hormone responsible for releasing stored fat) from entering the blood stream.

Therefore, simple sugars have two negative effects against weight loss: they promote fat storage and hinder fat release.

41. Be cool, lose weight.

Just as being hot burns up calories, being cool does, too. (Being cool also helps the mind to work more effectively. Sixty degrees is good for thinking.)

42. *Fiber is filling.*

Foods with fiber will help to fill you up and you can then avoid higher-calorie foods.

Soluble fiber (e.g., oat bran) will lower your cholesterol; insoluble fiber (e.g., wheat bran) will be good for your intestines and help prevent colon cancer.

43. *Life does begin again.*

Everything is different, much better, when you become slim.

By the way, sit-ups do not reduce your weight around your middle (there is no such thing as spot reducing), but they do tone and firm the area.

44. Move it!

Park your car far away from the mall, your work place, etc., and walk. Walk briskly through the house, everywhere. Move around.

Always take the stairs, if you can. (I think it works better for weight loss than stepper machines.)

Walk, run, jog, move!

Brisk walking, jogging and running are all good exercises for weight loss. Be as active as you can be, within your limits.

There are many books, magazines and videos available on these exercises. Investigate them for whichever of these exercises you choose to do to learn more about techniques and to get the maximum benefit.

45. Bagels are low-fat —and filling, too!

Some plain or onion bagels have only 150 calories each. But read the label! Some have more calories. (Personally, I believe that bagels feed the soul as well as the body!)

46. Spice is nice!

It will help you to eat many cucumbers, lettuce, carrots, etc.

Don't use salt unless you need to. There is sodium in bread, veggies, etc. With conflicting research reports on salt intake, you should be guided by your own health counselor's appraisal of your personal needs.

Salt tends to retain fluid (means more weight). Also, you might avoid celery. Although it is nearly calorie-free, it has much sodium.

47. Remember to pray.

Ask for aid in losing weight. It really will help. Pray, and believe that you will lose weight.

48. Bored? Do anything but eat!

Don't eat when bored, lonely, nervous, anxious, depressed or just because it's lunch time, etc.

Eat when you are truly hungry, because your body actually needs food. But eat low-calorie and low-fat foods.

When you aren't really hungry but have an impulse to eat anyway, take a brisk walk instead—call a friend, sing, write a poem, read, clean a room.

Do anything but eat!!!

49. *Never buy a size larger!*

Never!
Don't give in!
Lose weight!

This "not buying a size larger" is important, because it means you're not letting the weight problem win!

50. *Think, dream about being slim.*

Think about how much you really want to lose weight.

Dream of the day you will have reached your goal.

Motivate yourself. You can lose weight!

51. *Beware of false hunger!*

A funny feeling in the stomach, perhaps nervousness or acid in the stomach, does not mean you are hungry.

Wait five minutes, or ten.

Drink a cup of coffee or herbal tea, eat a raw carrot, or brush your teeth. (Helps a lot!)

The false hunger will go away.

52. *You can lose weight—IF.*

If you follow all the instructions here—all that fit your circumstances and physical abilities. Remember how I did it: no animal foods (meat, poultry, fish); no animal products (eggs and dairy products). Exercise.

Look again at "Some good advice about food choices" for guidance on this kind of diet (Page 11), and do consult your own health counselor.

53. *Say 'WHEN I lose weight, WHEN I'm slim.' Not 'IF.'*

Confident, upbeat, positive thinking really helps!

54. Total calories do count.

When dieting, the most important calorie count is the number of calories from fat, but it is also important to know the total number of calories (at least approximately) in each serving of food you eat.

Here's a list that puts things in perspective. It shows that it's not so much the amount you eat but more what you eat that puts on the extra weight.

This list also shows that you don't have to be hungry while you are losing weight.

There are the same number of calories in . . .

> 1 tablespoon of peanut butter or 20 cups of lentil sprouts.

> 1 cup of whole milk or 20 cups of steamed
>   spinach.
> 3 cheese enchiladas or 200 cups of cooked collard
>   greens.
> 1 chocolate bar or 15 cups of raspberries

For lots more such comparisons, see Susan Powter's book, *Stop the Insanity.* New York: Pocket Books, pp. 144-147.

55. Lean, red meat? Ha!

Dr. Neal Barnard (*Food for Life.* New York: Crown), explains that although the fat you can see can be trimmed off of meat, it is impossible to remove the fat that permeates the meat. Ground beef is about 60 percent fat. Extra-lean ground beef is 54 percent fat, top loin is 40 percent fat, round tip is 36 percent fat and top round is 29 percent fat. "'Lean meat,' is a contradiction in terms."

56. *Losing weight is simple . . . honestly.*

Choose low-calorie, low-fat, healthful food.
Increase your metabolic rate.
Exercise, exercise, exercise.
That's it.
That's all.

57. *Banish fattening foods.*

Be sure to get rid of all the fattening foods in the house. They are probably over-processed and un-healthful even for any slim people who might be around.

Mark Victor Hansen and Jack Canfield are right on target when they tell you to start your diet in the supermarket. If you don't buy it you can't eat it, they say.

One thing I think you should buy is mustard. It has less than five calories per serving. I used Gulden's Spicy Brown Mustard. It was great help for me— because . . .

I used it:

- instead of jelly on toast
- instead of butter or margarine on baked potatoes
- on salad for salad dressing
- on low fat crackers
- on the raw onions (delicious!) in my raw onion-on-whole-wheat sandwich
- on veggies instead of butter or margarine
- to flavor just about everything!

Of course, if you prefer the yellow un-spicy mustard, that also comes in a zero-calories type. (Just let me say—if any of the folks at Gulden's want me to do a commercial, I'm ready!) But let me add this: some folks may be somewhat allergic to mustard. Sorry.

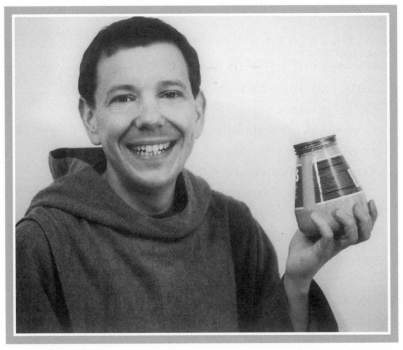

Not kidding a bit—a perky product like mustard can be a saving savor in a diet!

Maybe you can find something like it, with just as few calories, that will add zip to some of the foods you eat.

58. Water, water, water.

Drink at least eight glasses (8 ounces each) of water every day. It is good for your health, helps you eat less and can take away false hunger.

59. There's no real joy in being fat.

Fat people aren't jolly. It's just that jolly people may tend to become fat!

But here's a "jolly" tofu recipe for you!

Scrambled Tofu

- 2 packages of low-fat tofu (Mori is a good brand)
- ½ cup finely chopped raw onion
- ½ cup chopped bell pepper
- 1 tablespoon curry powder (or less if you prefer)
- 2 slices of whole wheat bread, finely crumbled

Mix all together, moisten a bit (if needed) with tomato or vegetable juice. Serve as a main course, with a salad or spread on diet whole wheat bread for a sandwich. Should be enough for three servings.

60. Call it fat!

Don't say you're overweight, chubby, plump, stout or obese.

Say fat.

And hate it (the fat, not yourself). You are a slim person inside trying to get out.

You can do it!

61. Exercise can reduce hunger.

It's my experience that moderate exercise actually reduces my hunger!

I find this true of exercises that warm the body such as walking, jogging, etc. But sports done out in winter's cold weather can increase my hunger.

Just for encouragement—walking briskly for 30 minutes burns 120 calories, a jog for 30 minutes burns 284 calories. If that is something you can do, get moving!

62. Skip exercise today; it will be easier to skip it tomorrow.

"I'll exercise tomorrow or later" is just wishful thinking, meaning you wish you didn't have to exercise!

Just remember that every move you make burns some calories.

The more you move the more you burn.

Also, exercise increases your metabolic rate. Cliff Sheats believes that you get the greatest fat-burning effect through aerobic exercise several times a week, if you are able to—45-60 minutes at a time.

Inactivity causes your muscles to waste away— and muscles burn calories.

63. Get plenty of sleep!

When you're tired you'll eat more, and you will also avoid exercising.

64. Here's a great cookbook:

Read *The Oats, Peas, Beans & Barley Cookbook*, by Edyth Young Cottrell (Santa Barbara, CA: Woodbridge Press).

It has many excellent recipes, some using soybeans

soybeans including soybean concentrate (replaces milk and eggs in many recipes) soy milk, soy cream, soy whipped topping and soy sour cream. (Together with recipes for making your own soybean concentrate and tofu, if you wish.)

65. Gallstones and fat.

A high-fat diet can cause gallstones, according to the findings of the famous Framingham (Massachusetts) Heart Study. So everyone, not just those who are overweight, should eat a low-fat diet.

66. *Look it up.*

Get a book that lists the fat content of various foods.

There is no such thing as meat, poultry, fish that is truly lean (Yes, I'm repeating—I thought you might not yet be convinced.)

In *Safe Foods*, by Dr. Michael F. Jacobson (New York: Berkley), you will learn that lean or even extra-lean ground beef have more than half of their calories in fat.

67. *Never go off your diet or miss your exercise.*

(Except for sickness.) But if you do, then go right back! Now! Not next Monday. Don't feel guilty. Just do it. Regain and keep up your momentum.

And please don't eat *because* you broke your diet!!!

68. *Look it up again.*

Buy a copy of *The Complete Book of Food Counts*, by Corinne T. Netzer (New York: Dell). It tells you the calories and fat content of many foods.

69. Meditate.

Think about why you are trying to lose weight. Focus—proceed in your thoughts to the glorious wonders of slimness. Think of becoming healthier for those you love. They need you, and they want you to be healthy.

70. Do more than 'look it up' —take it with you.

Go to the store with your calorie and fat book or chart.

Find and buy interesting, low calorie foods. Strive for more variety in healthful foods.

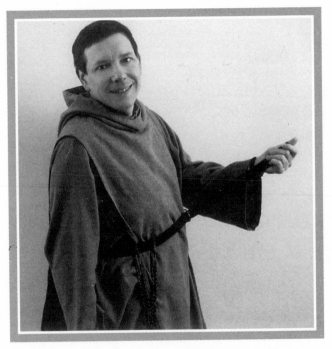

Sublime happiness is watching those inches melt away!

71. Ignore all the 'good cheer' talk about fat.

Being fat is lousy, miserable, rotten and unhealthy. Ignore those talk shows where people say, "We make too much of being slim in this country. You have to accept yourself."

But you don't have to accept excessive fat. Such fat is dangerous. Don't accept a condition that could lead to a heart attack, stroke or cancer.

72. Gout? Sure.

Overweight and/or a high-fat diet can cause some people to be more prone to gout. What is gout? Painful inflammation of the joints, especially those of hands and feet. You don't want it.

73. Laugh and feel good.

Keep and increase your sense of humor. It will help. Laughter, especially big laughs, burns up calories! As Miss Piggy says, "Never eat more than you can lift."

74. Lose weight in the water.

Swimming doesn't burn up many calories, unless you do many laps. (Try it, if you can.)

Stretching in the water is great fun.

Aerobics in the water (*e.g.*, jogging in place) is an excellent fat-burning exercise.

75. Get steamed.

Saunas, steam baths burn up a few calories. (They also release fluids.)

Mostly they'll loosen you up to exercise and make you feel great, without calories. They'll invigorate you, give you a positive attitude and a greater desire to exercise, to be slim and healthy.

76. Dine with style.

When you eat, prepare everything well. Sit down, relax, eat very slowly and chew everything a lot.

Add candles, music, etc., rather than adding something to your plate.

And do put the food on a plate. Never eat out of a container, which can lead to eating too much.

Know (about) how many calories are in everything you eat.

77. *Look around;*
make comparisons.

Look at other overweight people. Tell yourself you don't want to be like that. Look at slim people. Tell yourself you do want to be like that.

78. *God wants you to be healthy.*
He really does.

God doesn't want us to be unhealthy. He wants us to live healthy, vibrant, youthful lives—to me, and I hope to you, that means slim and fit!

79. *Stand up for slimness.*

Standing burns more calories than sitting; walking more than standing.

And, while you're standing . . . why not make yourself a great salad!

A great low-calorie, fat-free salad that I enjoy very often consists of green-leaf lettuce, raw spinach, raw onions, carrots, mushrooms, radishes and tomatoes.

Sometimes I top it with bean or seed sprouts. For dressing I use spicy brown mustard or cold tomato sauce. Please believe me, these "dressings" are much better than they sound!

80. Just 'thinking thin' won't do it.

Yes, "think thin," but let that make you diet and exercise. Thinking alone doesn't work.

81. Be thankful for a reality check.

Thank all the people who have told (or tell) you that you are fat.

They care. I'm grateful for all the lousy, wonderful, rotten, encouraging things people said to me! Thanks, folks.

82. Love your world of water.

Drink water, coffee, tea, herbal tea and more water. Avoid soda, fruit juice (eat fruit—less sugar, more filling).

83. Select exclusively 'slim snacks.'

Practice saying that's what you are going to do, and be determined to eat something like the items listed below when hungry:

- Raw carrots
- Lettuce
- Radishes
- Raw onions
- Scallions

84. Get it off your chest!

Overweight with much fat on the chest causes lung and diaphragm movement to be impaired. This strains the heart. It also aggravates any respiratory problems.

85. *Avoid fake diets.*

Like these:

1. Losing weight fast. (About two pounds a week is a good rate.)
2. Eat what you want, just think thin. (Doesn't work.)
3. Purge yourself. (Never make yourself vomit no matter how many excess calories you have eaten. Please don't, I love you.)

86. Don't expect pasta to make you thin.

Years ago dieters avoided pasta. Now they are encouraged to eat it. Which is correct?

There are 210 calories in half a cup of uncooked pasta. That's enough, when cooked, to make about a couple of handfuls.

Does anyone eat that little pasta?

It is too high in calories and too low in nutrients (if not made from a whole grain) to be part of your diet. Sorry.

87. Read, don't feed. Books can improve your looks. Honestly.

What I'm going to suggest here is perhaps my most original (or unusual) contribution to the world of weight loss.

It is another great way to deal with false hunger, which I believe is a very real cause of over-eating.

My suggestion is this: when false hunger strikes or you feel like eating but are not really hungry—read a good book. Choose one that so engages your interest that it takes your mind off your hunger.

It really helps.

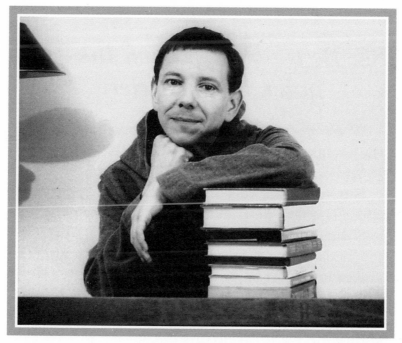

Reading can help you to suppress false hunger.
While losing 114 pounds I read a <u>lot</u> of books!

88. Be tough. Get past the 'quick loss' barrier.

When you begin a diet and exercise program the weight comes off rather quickly at first.

You're losing some fat and lots of water.

But get closer to your goal, and it's tough to lose those last few pounds.

Solution—you get tougher!

Check to see if you are cutting out as many calories and as much fat as you can, healthfully.

And exercise more. If your fitness has been improving and you can exercise more, safely, it should help a lot in losing those last, difficult pounds.

89. *Fat = Unhealthy. Fit = Healthy.*

As you lose fat your body will be fitter, healthier. You'll even sleep better. Best of all you'll burn up more fat. Your metabolic rate increases the more fit you become.

90. *Do not starve yourself.*

You don't need to starve. That's unhealthful and actually slows down the metabolic rate, causing you to burn up fewer calories.

According to Dr. Neal Barnard, body fat is the body's "fuel reserve," and starvation turns down the thermostat, so to speak, to conserve fuel until the starvation is over.

If you're overweight, your body will use up muscle, not fat.

On this program you don't ever have to be hungry to lose weight ("Here he goes again!"): raw carrots, cucumbers, lettuce, pickles, diet whole wheat bread . . .

And please remember, potatoes are not a high-calorie food.

91. Baking without shortening?

Applesauce!

You can indeed make your baking lower in fat and calories by using unsweetened applesauce instead of shortening or oil.

I've done this with excellent results.

Use the same amount of applesauce as you would shortening or oil, according to the recipe.

92. Don't pressure your stomach.

Excess weight around the abdomen puts pressure on the stomach. That can force acid back up the esophagus, causing heartburn.

93. Let's say it again: don't skip breakfast!

That's a bad way to diet. You'll probably eat more (too much) later if you skip breakfast.

However, breakfast doesn't have to be the minute you get up. It can be a little later.

Don't feel hungry in the morning? I know why!

Adele Davis gave the answer years ago—you probably ate too much the night before!

But don't let too much time go by before having breakfast. Don't wait until you're very hungry to eat—if you do you might (probably? will?) eat the wrong things and too much of them.

94. Don't lie to yourself.

Lies overweight people love:

1. "I can't help it, my mother was overweight. It runs in the family." Heredity may be a fat-factor but it's still possible to lose weight if you really try.

2. "I've tried every diet. They don't work." Good diets work. This one works.

3. "I eat so little." This is a half-truth lie.

Many slim people can out-eat overweight people. Slim, fit people have healthy appetites.

Fat people have tired bodies and tired appetites. They eat because they feel weak and tired. They feel weak and are tired because they are overweight. They're overweight because of what they eat. They

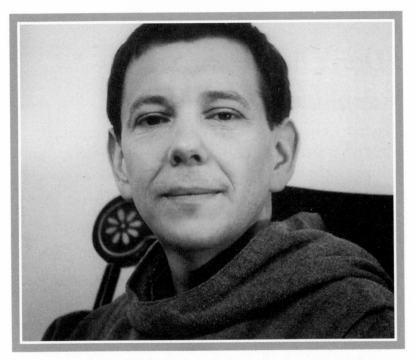

It's wrong to tell a lie!

say they eat so little. But what do they eat too often? Potato chips, soda, pizza, cake, etc.? Ignore your taste buds!

4. "I can't exercise; I don't have time. It hurts, or I'm too overweight." You have to, you have to, you have to.

5. "I'll only gain the weight back."

If you go off your diet, of course you will. If you want to stay slim, after you reach your goal continue to exercise and then you can safely take in some more calories—still watching the fat content.

6. "I'm nice; who cares what I weigh?"

You are nice. I care. Lose weight. It will make you healthier and happier.

95. *Reality check, again.*

When I was overweight someone noticed me reading a book, resting the book on the "shelf" below my chest! (Actually it was a kind of a two-step arrangement of fat.)

Also, a kid once actually tried to set a small plate on it, saying, "I'll put it here."

96. *Be sure to drink plenty of liquids.*

Dehydration is more common than people realize. Having suffered from it myself, I can tell you that it's no fun. Drink at least eight ounces of water eight times a day. Don't wait until you are thirsty!

97. *Here are three excellent books.*

The first two provide convincing information on why a vegan diet is the healthiest one, even for people who are not overweight. Both are by John Robbins:

Diet for a New America tells "how your food choices affect your health, happiness and the future of life on earth" (Walpole, NH: Stillpoint).

May All Be Fed deals with health issues and food lobbies, and includes excellent recipes by Jia Patton and others (New York: William Morrow).

Also, there's a vegan cookbook, *Vegan Delights—Gourmet Vegan Specialties*, by Jeanne Marie Martin. (Madeira Park, BC, Canada: Harbour.)

98. Exercise revives energy.

Often tiredness is the excuse given for not exercising. Yet exercising really perks up a tired body and a tired mind.

Feeling tired? Get going! Get exercising! You'll feel totally revived!

99. Read this book, often.

Leaf through it every day.

Let it be my pep talk to you personally, to help you lose weight!

100. You CAN lose weight!

Love Yourself, so . . .
HATE THE WEIGHT!!!

P.S. This program really works. I'm proof. In fact, when I got down to 123 pounds, some people thought it had worked too well (I'm 5'7"). People thought my face looked gaunt. Three friends didn't even recognize me. One actually asked my name. (No kidding!) One friend even needed some convincing.

Many people (even strangers) asked if I was sick. At first I loved it! Then it got tiring. So I started wearing an "I'm not sick" sign. (Kidding.) Since people were really concerned—a couple of them even cried—I decided to gain weight!!! Can you believe it?

Since I wouldn't eat cholesterol, saturated fat, animals or animal products, it was slow. (Does seem to prove my point—that those foods make a person fat.) I even joked about standing on my head while eating, so the calories would go to my face.

Finally, I regained 25 pounds, making me 148 pounds (Some of it *muscle* from weight lifting!)

Now, people think I look healthy. (See my "after" photo on the back cover.)

But since I don't want to gain back any more weight I have to be very careful of what I eat. And I'm careful to keep exercising, lifting weights, watching what I eat—so that my now 148 pounds won't become 158, 168 . . .

About the Author

Brother Craig is a Catholic monk, founder of The Monks of Adoration, in Petersham, Massachusetts.

He has written five books, including *The Coming Chastisement* which made the Catholic bestseller list, as well as a play and several short stories. He also writes poetry and enjoys studying the life and work of Emily Dickinson.

Brother Craig writes six columns, including *Health and Nutrition*, for various publications.

Born in Boston, he studied acting as a youth and won several acting awards. He lived and studied in Ireland before beginning his B.A. in religious studies at the University of Albuquerque. He completed

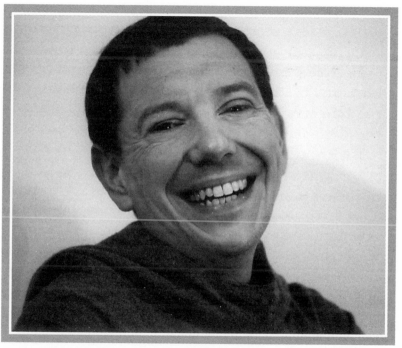

Believe me, a thinner, healthier body <u>will</u> make you happy—very happy!

college in six semesters; did 35 credit hours during his last semester and graduated *magna cum laude*.

He received his B.A. in philosophy, and his B.A., M.A. and S.T.L. (Licentiate in Sacred Theology) from the University of Saint Thomas Aquinas in Rome, the alma mater of Pope John Paul II.

Brother Craig is a popular, enthusiastic (and very entertaining) speaker at conferences, where he gives uplifting motivational talks.

For information regarding *Love Yourself, so . . . Hate the Weight!* seminars or for speaking engagements, contact:

The Monks of Adoration, Post Office Box 546, Petersham, MA 01366-0546. Phone (508) 724-8871.

For e-mail: Catholic_Monks_of_Adoration@Compuserve.com, or see their homepage at: http://www.rc.net/org/monks.

References

Bailey, Covert and Lea Bishop. *The Fit or Fat Woman*. Boston: Houghton Mifflin, 1989. (215 Park Ave., New York, NY 10003)

Barnard, Neal. *Foods That Cause You To Lose Weight — The Negative Calorie Effect*. McKinney, Texas: The Magni Group, 1992. (P. O. Box 849, McKinney TX 75070)

Barnard, Neal. *Food for Life*. New York: Crown, 1993. (201 East 50th St., New York, NY 10022)

The Catholic Truth Society. *The Holy Bible, Revised Standard Edition (Catholic Edition)*. London, 1952. (38-40 Eccleston Square, London, England SW2)

Canfield, Jack and Mark Victor Hansen. *Dare to Win*. New York: Berkley Books, 1996. (200 Madison Ave., New York, NY 10016)

Cottrell, Edyth Young. *The Oats, Peas, Beans and Barley Cookbook*. Santa Barbara, CA: Woodbridge Press, 1982. (P. O. Box 209, Santa Barbara, CA 93102)

Jackowski, Edward J. *Hold It! You're Exercising Wrong!* New York: Fireside, 1995. (1230 Avenue of the Americas, New York, NY 10020)

Jacobson, Michael F., *et.al. Safe Foods.* New York: Berkley, 1991.
(200 Madison Ave., New York, NY 10016)

Klapper, Michael. *Vegan Nutrition: Pure and Simple.* Umatilla, FL: Gentle
World. (P. O. Box 1418, Umatilla, FL 32784)

Martin, Jeanne Marie. *Vegan Delights—Gourmet Vegan Specialties.*
Madeira Park, B.C.: Harbour, 1993. (P. O. Box 219, Madeira Park, BC
Canada V0N 2H0.

Mindell, Earl. *Earl Mindell's Live Longer and Feel Better with Vitamins
and Minerals.* New Canaan, CT: Keats Publishing, 1994. (P.O. Box 876,
New Canaan, CT 06840-0876)

Natow, Annette B. and Jo-Ann Heslin. *The Fat Attack.* New York: Pocket
Books, 1990. (1230 Avenue of the Americas, New York, NY 10020)

Netzer, Corinne T. *The Complete Book of Food Counts.* New York: Dell,
1994. (Bantam, Doubleday, Dell, 1540 Broadway, New York, NY
10036)

Null, Gary and Steve Null. *The Complete Handbook of Nutrition.* New
York: Houghton Mifflin, 1972. (1540 Broadway, New York, NY 10036)

Ornish, Dean. *Dr. Dean Ornish's Program for Reversing Heart Disease.*
New York: Ivy Books, 1991. (Ballantine Books: 201 E. 50th St., New
York, NY 10022)

Ornish, Dean. *Eat More, Weigh Less*. New York: HarperCollins, 1993.
(10 East 53rd St., New York, NY 10022)

Powter, Susan. *Stop the Insanity*. New York: Pocket Books, 1993. (1230
Avenue of the Americas, New York, NY 10020)

Robbins, John. *Diet for a New America*. Walpole, NH: Stillpoint Publishing, 1987. (P. O. Box 640, Walpole, N.H. 03608-0640)

Robbins, John. *May All Be Fed*. New York: William Morrow, 1992. (1350
Avenue of the Americas, New York, NY 10019)

Scott, David. *David Scott's Protein-Balanced Cookery*. Sebastopol, CA:
CRCS Publications, 1987. (P. O. Box 1460, Sebastopol, CA 95472)

Sheats, Cliff. *Cliff Sheat's Lean Bodies*. New York: Warner Books, 1995.
(1271 Avenue of the Americas, New York, NY 10020)

Time-Life Books. *Staying Flexible—The Full Range of Motion*. Alexandria,
VA: Time-Life Books, 1987. (777 Duke St., Alexandria, VA 22314)

Weil, Andrew. *Natural Health, Natural Medicine*. New York: Houghton
Mifflin. (215 Park Ave., New York, NY 10003)